CONSTIPA~~~~

CURES

The Ugly Fact About Chronic Constipation and How to Kick It Off Naturally

James Edwards

TABLE OF CONTENTS

INTRODUCTION

In a world where busy programs and fast-paced lifestyles rule our everyday routines, millions of people suffer from the silent battle of chronic constipation, which has a subtle but profound effect on those who experience its discomfort. This condition's chronicity not only has a devastating effect on physical health but also lowers overall quality of life. It's becoming more and more clear as we make our way through the maze of contemporary life that finding true health and vitality frequently originates from within, and for many, that path starts with attaining ideal digestive balance.

Welcome to 'CONSTIPATION CURES', a thorough guide devoted to revealing the secrets of persistent constipation and offering a path to alleviation naturally. We set out on a journey in these pages that goes beyond the constraints of makeshift and short-term fixes. Rather, we investigate the underlying causes of digestive dysregulation and the complex network of variables that lead to persistent constipation. This book promotes a transformative strategy that looks at the digestive system as a whole, addressing the symptoms as well as trying to bring it back into balance.

You will gain valuable knowledge, evidence-based tactics, and useful advice as we go through the chapters, giving you the ability to take charge of your digestive health. With advice on everything from diet and lifestyle changes to natural remedy research, 'CONSTIPATION CURES' wants to be your go-to guide for long-lasting comfort. This book aims to close the knowledge gap between traditional medicine and modern science by incorporating the wisdom of healing traditions and the most recent developments in medical science.

'CONSTIPATION CURES' is intended to serve as a source of hope and information, regardless of whether you have been fighting chronic constipation for years or are just trying to strengthen your digestive resilience. Together, let's set out to live a life free from the confines of persistent constipation, where good digestive health is equated with overall well-being. This book is your key to unlocking the ability to naturally change the course of your digestive destiny and kick off chronic constipation.

CHAPTER ONE

Mastering Chronic Constipation

Chronic constipation is a widespread gastrointestinal problem that millions of people experience globally. Constipation is a common occurrence, but persistent and protracted problems with bowel movements can have a serious negative influence on one's quality of life. This chapter attempts to give readers a thorough understanding of the definition and underlying causes of chronic constipation.

The meaning of chronic constipation

Occassional bowel movements, difficulty passing stools, or a feeling of incomplete evacuation are the hallmarks of chronic constipation. When these symptoms last for more than three months, or for an extended period of time, the condition is usually diagnosed. People who suffer from long-term constipation may also feel uncomfortable, bloated, or have abdominal pain, which can further impair their general health.

Causes of Chronic Constipation

1. Nutritional Elements:

a. Low Intake of Fiber: Constipation may result from a diet low in fiber. Fiber gives stools more volume, which facilitates passage. One of the most common causes of chronic constipation is inadequate fiber intake.

CHAPTER TWO

Effects of Natural Remedies of Constipation on Well-Being and Life Quality

Efforts to naturally kick off chronic constipation have a significant impact on general health and quality of life. Investigating the holistic methods and way of life adjustments that help with this prevalent condition reveals a series of advantages that go well beyond the quick alleviation of constipation. This chapter delves into the ways in which gut health, general well-being, and the transformative path to optimal health are interdependent.

The Relationship Between the Stomach and the Body

The human gut is frequently referred to as the "second brain" because of its intricate neuronal network and capacity to affect a range of physiological processes. This delicate balance is upset by persistent constipation, which has a declining effect on general health. By treating constipation naturally, we also support the complex network of connections that exist between the gastrointestinal tract and the body as a whole.

1. Better Digestive Function:

a. Dietary changes and the addition of foods high in fiber facilitate more easily digested food.

b. Probiotics support the best possible digestive function by helping to maintain a balanced gut microbiome.

2. Improved Nutrient Absorption: A gut that is in good health makes it easier for vital nutrients to be absorbed, which promotes general wellness.

3. Enhanced Immune System: A healthy gut helps to maintain a strong immune system, which protects the body from diseases and infections.

Increasing Vitality

People who experience chronic constipation frequently experience exhaustion and depletion. When people use natural remedies and address the underlying causes, their energy levels are revitalized, which has a substantial impact on their day-to-day lives.

1. Balanced Hormones: Consistent bowel movements help maintain hormonal balance, which lowers fatigue and increases energy levels that last all day.

2. Better Quality of Sleep: Having a healthy gut rhythm can have a beneficial impact on sleep cycles, resulting in more rejuvenating and restorative sleep.

Emotional and Mental Health

The gut-brain axis is important for mental health, and stress, anxiety, and discomfort can all be exacerbated by chronic constipation. We can unleash the potential for better mental and emotional health by naturally treating constipation.

1. Lower Stress Levels: Holistic methods, like mindful eating and stress-reduction exercises, help to lower overall stress by calming the nervous system.

2. Improved Mood: Neurotransmitter production is positively influenced by a healthy gut, which supports emotional stability and a balanced mood.

3. Enhanced Cognitive Function: Better digestion and nutrient absorption support improved cognitive function, which in turn supports sharper thinking and mental acuity.

Changes in Life Quality

Physical relief is only one aspect of using natural remedies to end chronic constipation. It acts as a catalyst for a comprehensive change that gives people the power to take back control of their health and well-being.

1. Enhanced Vitality: Enhanced energy, better digestion, and regular bowel movements all add to a general feeling of vigor and vitality.

2. Empowerment Through Knowledge: By embracing natural remedies and being aware of the body's needs, people can feel more empowered and take an active role in their own health journey.

In summary, we observe a significant impact on health and quality of life as we work toward naturally curing chronic constipation. This journey is about laying the groundwork for holistic well-being rather than just treating a single symptom. Through nourishing the gut-body connection, replenishing energy, and fostering mental and emotional equilibrium, people set out on a life-changing path towards optimum health and a vibrant, joyful existence.

CHAPTER THREE

The Importance of Natural Remedies

It's simple to lose touch with the natural cycles and processes that regulate our well-being in the hectic, modern lives we lead. Digestion is one such vital process that is frequently taken for granted. When it malfunctions, as it can in the case of chronic constipation, it can significantly affect our general health and quality of life. This chapter explores the need for natural remedies to deal with chronic constipation and how accepting the wisdom of nature can offer long-lasting relief.

The Current Puzzle

The emergence of processed foods, sedentary lifestyles, and high levels of stress are all major contributors to the rise in chronic constipation in our modern world. Processed foods are deficient in the fiber required for healthy digestion, and our increasingly sedentary lifestyles prevent the natural movement that encourages regular bowel movements. Many people consequently discover themselves caught in a loop of discomfort and annoyance.

The Disadvantage of Orthodox Medicine

Pharmaceutical interventions are widely accessible, but they may only offer momentary relief and frequently have a variety of side effects. For example, using laxatives excessively can cause dependency and further interfere with the digestive system's normal operation. Using natural remedies becomes essential as we work toward a more sustainable and comprehensive approach to health.

CHAPTER FOUR

Deciphering the Digestive System's Function

The digestive system is a key player in the complex orchestra of our bodies. It conducts a symphony of processes that convert food into the nutrients our bodies require to function at their best. Understanding the complex workings of the digestive system is essential to naturally curing chronic constipation. The main elements of the digestive system will be covered in detail in this chapter, along with how they support bowel regularity and help avoid constipation.

The Essential Parts of the Digestive System

The digestive system is made up of multiple organs that cooperate to process food, absorb nutrients, and eliminate waste. Let's examine these different organs in brief detail:

1. Mouth: The Intro of Digestion

Food is first broken down into smaller pieces in the mouth during the mastication process, which starts the digestive process. In addition to aiding in digestion, chewing causes the release of enzymes like amylase, which accelerates the breakdown of carbohydrates.

2. The Stomach:

During the digestive process, the stomach plays a major role by secreting acids and gastric juices that help break down the food even more. In addition to facilitating digestion, this acidic environment sanitizes the food that has been consumed, shielding the body from dangerous bacteria and infections.

3. The Small Intestine: The Epicenter of Digestion

It is in the small intestine that most nutrients are absorbed. The breakdown of food is further facilitated by the bile from the liver and the pancreas, which allows essential nutrients to enter the bloodstream. The body's tissues and cells are then nourished by this nutrient-rich blood.

4. Large Intestine:

Water and electrolytes are reabsorbed as the digested remains to pass into the large intestine and form stool. The gut microbiota, which is made up of trillions of bacteria, is found in the large intestine. The fermentation of undigested carbohydrates by this microbial community results in short-chain fatty acids, which support regular bowel movements.

The Melodic Beat of Peristalsis

The rhythm section of our digestive symphony is similar to peristalsis, the coordinated muscle contractions that move food through the digestive tract. Food must pass easily from the esophagus to the rectum in order for regular bowel movements to occur, which is ensured by proper peristalsis.

Hydration:

In order to keep the digestive process fluid, water acts as the conductor of the digestive flow. Dehydration can cause hard, dry stools, which are a common sign of constipation. Maintaining proper hydration encourages the softening of stool, which facilitates easier passage through the intestines.

The Brain-Gut Relationship

The gut-brain axis facilitates close communication between the brain and the digestive system. Digestion can be impacted by psychological and emotional factors. Tension, stress, and anxiety can all cause constipation by interfering with the digestive system's regular operation. Deep breathing exercises and relaxation methods are examples of mindful practices that can ease the gut-brain connection and support a healthy digestive system.

In conclusion, kicking off chronic constipation naturally requires an understanding of the digestive system's harmonical operation. Through mindful practices, appropriate hydration, and nutrition, you can support the harmonious performance of your digestive flow, encouraging regular bowel movements and general well-being. We'll look at dietary and lifestyle approaches to help maintain a healthy digestive system and say goodbye to chronic constipation in the upcoming chapter.

CHAPTER FIVE

Understanding the Impact of Gut Health on Constipation

It is critical to investigate the complex relationship between gut health and the commonness of constipation in the quest to eliminate chronic constipation naturally. The digestive system is a complex network of organs, and the gut, also known as the "second brain," plays an important role in overall health, including regular bowel movements. In this chapter, we look at the mechanisms that influence constipation and discuss natural ways to promote a healthy gut for better digestive function.

The Gut Microbiome: A Microorganism Symphony

The microbiome — a diverse community of trillions of microorganisms including bacteria, viruses, fungi, and other microbes — is at the heart of gut health. The gut's microbial community is essential for proper digestion, absorption of nutrients, and preservation of the intestinal lining. Constipation is one of the many digestive problems that can arise from upsetting this delicate ecosystem's balance.

Microbial Disproportion and Constipation

Constipation may be exacerbated by dysbiosis, an imbalance in the gut microbiome. Certain bacterial strains are essential for the synthesis of short-chain fatty acids, the breakdown of complex carbohydrates, and the encouragement of

CHAPTER SIX

Impact of Microbiome on Chronic Constipation

The microbiome, which is made up of trillions of microorganisms, is a complex ecosystem found in the human body. These microscopic residents have a significant impact on many body processes, such as digestion and gut health, and they are essential to preserving general health and well-being. The complex relationship between the microbiome and chronic constipation will be discussed in this chapter, along with how understanding and promoting this dynamic community can help reduce constipation naturally.

The Microbiome Revealed

The diverse community of bacteria, viruses, fungi, and other microorganisms that live in the gastrointestinal tract is referred to as the microbiome. These microscopic organisms support the immune system, break down complex carbohydrates, and synthesize vital vitamins, among many other tasks. Researchers have started to understand the profound influence of gut health and the microbiome in recent years.

Constipation and the Diversity of Microbiomes

Diversity, or the existence of a large variety of microbial species, is a hallmark of a healthy gut microbiome. According to studies, people who experience chronic constipation frequently have less variety of microorganisms in their gut.

Constipation may result from this dysbiosis, an imbalance that impairs the effectiveness of the digestive system.

Gut Bacteria's Function in Digestion

A few specific gut bacterial strains are essential for the digestion of dietary fiber. Fiber, which can be found in whole grains, fruits, and vegetables, is crucial for encouraging regular bowel movements. As a byproduct of fermentation, gut bacteria produce short-chain fatty acids (SCFAs) from the fiber. In addition to improving water absorption and stimulating muscular contractions, SCFAs also feed the cells that line the colon, all of which support regular bowel movements.

Probiotics and Constipation Alleviation

Live beneficial bacteria, or probiotics, have been shown to be helpful in preserving a balanced microbiome. Supplements and fermented foods such as yogurt, kefir, and sauerkraut are good sources of these microorganisms. It has been demonstrated that probiotics alter the gut microbiome, encouraging a more diverse and well-balanced bacterial community. Certain probiotic strains, like Lactobacillus and Bifidobacterium, may be especially helpful for relieving constipation, according to research.

Prebiotics to Promote Gut Health

Prebiotics are indigestible fibers that feed good bacteria in the gut. You can encourage the growth of these beneficial microbes by including prebiotic-rich foods in your diet, such as garlic, onions, bananas, and asparagus. This promotes optimal digestion by improving the general health of your microbiome.

Striking a Balance between Lifestyle and Microbiome

Although diet is very important, the microbiome is also influenced by other aspects of lifestyle. Stress, sleep deprivation, and sedentary lifestyles can all lead to dysbiosis in the gut flora. A comprehensive strategy for promoting a healthy microbiome and preventing chronic constipation must include stress-relieving activities, getting enough sleep, and engaging in regular physical activity.

In summary, a crucial first step toward obtaining long-lasting relief from chronic constipation is comprehending the complex interactions between the microbiome and the condition. Through a combination of dietary and lifestyle interventions, people can empower themselves to naturally eliminate constipation and cultivate long-lasting digestive health by nourishing and maintaining a diverse and balanced microbiome. We will explore doable tactics and all-natural solutions that leverage the microbiome's ability to support regular bowel movements and general health in the upcoming chapter.

CHAPTER SEVEN

Fiber: The Broom of Nature

Fiber, also known as "nature's broom," is one of the most powerful tools we have in our arsenal for kicking off chronic constipation naturally. This modest part of our diet is essential for preserving the health of our digestive tract and avoiding constipation.

Mastering Fiber

One kind of carbohydrate that the body is unable to process is fiber. Rather, it mostly makes its way through the digestive system undamaged, fulfilling a number of crucial roles in the process. Dietary fiber comes in two primary varieties: soluble and insoluble.

a. Soluble Fiber: This kind turns into a gel-like substance when it dissolves in water. It can assist in lowering blood sugar and cholesterol. Soluble fiber-containing foods include fruits, vegetables, beans, and oats.

b. Insoluble Fiber: This type of fiber does not dissolve in water, in contrast to soluble fiber. It helps the stool pass through the digestive system and gives it more volume. Nuts, whole grains, and a variety of vegetables are great providers of insoluble fiber.

Fiber's Function in Digestive Health

CHAPTER EIGHT

Water for Healthy Digestive System

Maintaining adequate hydration is essential for good health and is also critical for the proper functioning of the digestive system. Staying properly hydrated is essential if you want to naturally overcome chronic constipation. Water is necessary for many body functions, such as digestion and the passage of waste products through the intestines. This chapter will discuss the importance of staying hydrated for digestive health and offer helpful advice on how to maximize your water intake to prevent and treat chronic constipation.

Hydration's Critical Role in Digestive Health

1. Digestion tract lubrication

From the mouth to the rectum, water functions as a natural lubricant for the entire digestive system. Sufficient hydration softens stool, which facilitates the intestines' passage of waste through the digestive system. Constipation is less likely when smoother bowel movements are facilitated by this lubrication.

2. Avoiding Hydration Losses

Constipation can be exacerbated by dehydration because it causes the body to remove more water from the stool, which makes it more difficult to pass. By keeping your body's fluid levels in check, you can avoid dehydration and help the softening of your stool, which will encourage regular, comfortable bowel movements.

3. Enhanced Absorption of Nutrients

For the intestines to absorb nutrients as effectively as possible, proper hydration is necessary. Nutrients are absorbed into the bloodstream and passed through the digestive tract more quickly in a well-hydrated body. Regular bowel movements and overall digestive health are supported by this improved nutrient absorption.

Practical Advice on Drinking Water to Reduce Constipation

1. Stay Hydrated Throughout the Day

Make a conscious effort to stay hydrated throughout the day by drinking enough water. Although a minimum of eight 8-ounce glasses of water should be consumed in a day, each person's requirements may differ depending on their age, weight, and degree of activity. Keep a reusable water bottle with you to keep track of and reach your daily water intake targets.

2. Add Natural Flavors to Water

If you find plain water boring, try adding cucumber slices, mint leaves, or slices of citrus fruits (oranges, lemons, or limes). This can encourage you to drink more water throughout the day and make hydrating more enjoyable.

3. Give Water-Rich Foods Priority

Include foods that are high in water in your diet, such as fruits and vegetables. Oranges, cucumbers, celery, and watermelon are a few examples. These foods supply vital vitamins, minerals, and fiber that promote digestive health in addition to helping you stay hydrated overall.

4. Minimize Drinks That Dehydrate

Drinks that dehydrate the body, such as alcohol and caffeine-containing beverages, should be avoided as they may cause fluid loss. If you do drink these, make sure to increase your water intake to counteract their effects.

In summary, hydration is a key component of the all-natural strategy for curing chronic constipation. You can promote the lubrication of the digestive tract, avoid dehydration, and improve nutrient absorption by making adequate water intake a priority. Consistently following these useful hydration tips can help support regular bowel movements and preserve the health of your digestive system. Consistency is essential, so incorporating these routines into your everyday activities can help you find long-term relief from chronic constipation.

CHAPTER NINE

Adopting a Constipation-Free Way of Life

Changes in lifestyle are essential if one hopes to naturally eradicate chronic constipation. In addition to dietary modifications, establishing healthy routines can make a big difference in regular bowel movements and overall digestive wellness. We'll look at a number of lifestyle changes in this chapter that can help you on your path to a life free of constipation.

1. Drinking Routines:

Staying properly hydrated is essential for preserving digestive health. Stools become softer when wet, which facilitates passing. Make sure you consume eight 8-ounce glasses of water or more each day. To help your digestive system get going in the morning, try having a glass of warm water first thing.

2. Frequent Physical Activity:

By encouraging bowel motions and lowering the risk of constipation, exercise supports a healthy digestive system. It will be important for you to aim to get a minimum of thirty minutes of moderate exercise every day. Engaging in physical activities such as walking, jogging, yoga, or cycling can help maintain an active digestive system.

3. Create a Regular Schedule: Bowel Habits Are Important

Include foods like yogurt, kefir, sauerkraut, kimchi, and miso in your diet that are naturally fermented. These delectable foods can make a delightful addition to your meals and are high in probiotics.

2. Probiotic Supplements:

If getting adequate probiotics from food alone is difficult, think about taking premium probiotic supplements. Make sure there are enough live cultures in the supplement as well as a range of strains.

3. Consume Foods Rich in Prebiotics:

Eat foods like asparagus, bananas, onions, and garlic that are high in prebiotics. Probiotics in the gut require prebiotic nourishment in order to flourish.

In conclusion, probiotics are an important part of the natural strategy for kicking off chronic constipation. These beneficial bacteria play a vital role in maintaining gut health by balancing the microbiome, improving digestion, regulating the immune system, and generating vital SCFAs. Including foods and supplements high in probiotics in your daily routine can help you prevent digestive disorders and maintain a regular and healthy gut.

CHAPTER ELEVEN

Five Herbs with the Power to Kick Off Chronic Constipation Naturally

One's quality of life can be greatly impacted by chronic constipation, which can be a persistent and frustrating condition. Herbal remedies have been used for centuries to relieve constipation symptoms and encourage regular bowel movements, even though dietary and lifestyle changes are still very important in managing the condition. We'll look at five herbs in this chapter that are well-known for helping people with chronic constipation.

Aloe Vera

Succulent plants like aloe vera have long been used for therapeutic purposes. Its inner leaf gel is made up of substances with a slight laxative effect.

How to Utilize:

1. Aloe Vera Juice: Take one to two ounces per day of aloe vera juice. Make sure it doesn't contain aloin, a substance that can induce cramps and diarrhea.

2. Aloe Vera Gel: Take 1-2 tablespoons of aloe vera gel on an empty stomach, mixed with juice or water.

1. Psyllium Husk Powder: Consume 1-2 tablespoons of psyllium husk powder before meals, mixed with water or juice.

2. Psyllium Husk Capsules: Adhere to the product label's suggested dosage.

Remember to drink enough water when taking psyllium to avoid becoming dehydrated.

Ultimately, using these herbal remedies as part of your regular routine can help relieve chronic constipation in a natural and safe manner. But before using herbal remedies, you should exercise caution and see a doctor, particularly if you have underlying medical conditions or are on other medications. Moreover, a thorough strategy for naturally curing chronic constipation should include lifestyle modifications like eating a well-balanced diet, drinking plenty of water, and exercising frequently.

CHAPTER TWELVE

The Mind-Body Connection Towards Kicking Off Chronic Constipation Naturally

We must acknowledge the significant impact of the mind-body connection on our digestive health as we work to naturally end chronic constipation. The complex interactions that exist between our mental and physical health can have a substantial effect on how well our digestive systems work. This chapter delves into the communication channels between the mind and body, examining the functions of stress, emotions, and mindfulness in the treatment and prevention of chronic constipation.

1. Being Aware of the Gut-Brain Axis:

The gastrointestinal tract and the central nervous system communicate in both directions through the gut-brain axis. The brain, the gut's enteric nervous system (ENS), and the large population of microbes living in the digestive tract are all parts of this complex network. Chronic constipation is one of the digestive problems that can result from disruptions in this communication.

2. The Effects of Stress on Digestion:

Prolonged stress can be harmful to digestive health and may even be a factor in constipation. The fight-or-flight reaction is triggered in response to stress, which takes energy away from non-essential processes like digestion. Constipation may result from this slowing down bowel motions.

Methods for Reducing Stress:

Incorporating stress-reduction methods like yoga, meditation, and deep breathing can help soothe the nervous system and support regular bowel movements and optimal digestion.

3. Feelings and Digestive Wellbeing:

Both positive and negative emotions have the power to affect how food is absorbed. Constipation can result from physical manifestations of anxiety, depression, and unresolved emotional issues that impact the muscles in the digestive tract.

Keeping a Journal and Releasing Emotions:

A healthier emotional state and better digestive function can be achieved by keeping a journal to track emotional triggers and investigating techniques for releasing emotions, such as counseling or expressive therapies.

4. Mindful Eating and Mindfulness:

Being mindful requires paying attention to the present moment at all times, even when eating. By encouraging awareness of food selections, chewing patterns, and the body's signals of hunger and fullness, mindful eating can improve digestion.

Techniques for Mindful Eating:

A better relationship with food and regular bowel movements can be supported by practices like chewing food well, enjoying each bite, and listening to your body's signals.

5. Techniques for Biofeedback and Relaxation:

A therapeutic strategy called biofeedback assists patients in regaining voluntary control over their physiological processes, including digestion. To ease pelvic floor muscle tension and encourage regular bowel movements, biofeedback can be combined with relaxation methods like progressive muscle relaxation.

In summary, the key to naturally curing chronic constipation is to acknowledge and support the mind-body connection. Through the use of stress reduction techniques, emotional well-being approaches, mindfulness exercises, and biofeedback exploration, people can take charge of their own empowerment and experience long-lasting relief from constipation. The pursuit of ideal digestive health can be greatly aided by the balance between the mind and body.

Guidelines: Arrange mixed berries and granola on top of Greek yogurt, then top with honey.

b. Almond butter on sliced apples:

Ingredients: Almond butter and apple slices.

Guidelines: For a filling and high-fiber snack, spread almond butter on apple slices.

4. A meal to promote digestive harmony:

a. Quinoa and roasted vegetable grilled salmon:

Ingredients: Salmon fillets, quinoa, asparagus, zucchini, lemon juice, and garlic.

Guidelines: Serve cooked quinoa over grilled salmon and roasted veggies that have been tossed in olive oil, lemon, and garlic.

b. Stir-fried vegetables:

Ingredients: snap peas, broccoli, bell peppers, ginger, garlic, and soy sauce.

Guidelines: Stir-fry vegetables and tofu together with garlic, ginger, and soy sauce.

5. Drinks That Rehydrate and Detoxify:

a. Detox Ginger Lemon Tea:

Ingredients: honey, lemon juice, and fresh ginger.

Guidelines: Add honey and lemon juice, then steep grated ginger in hot water.

b. Mint and cucumber-infused water:

Ingredients: cucumber slices, water, and fresh mint leaves.

Guidelines: Mix water with cucumber and mint, then chill for a revitalizing drink.

In conclusion, these meal plans and recipes are meant to serve as a basis for a diet that promotes digestive health and aids in kicking off chronic constipation naturally. Always remember to drink plenty of water, eat a range of fruits and vegetables, and pay attention to your body's cues. For long-lasting effects, incorporate these recipes into your daily routine since consistency is essential.

CONCLUSION

The path to naturally kick off chronic constipation is a life-changing investigation of the complex interplay between diet, lifestyle, and general health. The goal of this book is to provide readers with the information and resources they need to overcome chronic stomach discomfort. Through exploring the domains of dietary modifications, mindful lifestyle, and holistic methods, we have discovered an abundance of techniques to cultivate a more robust gut and reestablish regularity.

We have learned the value of developing a healthy relationship with our bodies, paying attention to their signals, and making sustainable decisions that support digestive wellness through the pages of this book. From the profound benefits of eating foods high in fiber and staying hydrated to the reviving impacts of exercising and managing stress, every chapter acts as a springboard for living a life unrestricted by chronic constipation.

As we come to the end of this chapter, my genuine wish is that the information and suggestions you have found here will help you on your own path to better digestive health. Recall that we are incredibly resilient creatures and that adopting natural remedies and changing one's lifestyle can help overcome chronic constipation. Accept the ideas presented in this book, modify them to fit your particular situation, and set out on a journey to a life that is more vibrant and free. I hope and pray that you experience optimal digestive health and are free to enjoy every moment without having to deal with chronic constipation.

Printed in Great Britain
by Amazon

39468818R00030